Dirty Talk

An Innovative, Alluring, And Enjoyable Approach To
Engage In Intellectually Provocative Discussions With
Individuals Of Any Background

I0090060

*(How To Stimulate Your Partner's Desire Intimately And
Ignite Passion Through Seductive Verbal
Communication)*

Mickey Ruiz

TABLEO OF CONTENT

Explicit Communication Area 1 – Cultivate Sensual Atmosphere

In the initial Dirty Talk Zone, you will generate the palpable emotional anticipation associated with carnal longing. This tension can only be alleviated through engaging in a deeply intimate and fulfilling physical connection. This space is optimally established through written correspondence, telephonic conversation, or in-person interaction within a social gathering or public venue where a multitude of individuals are present.

Text messaging presents a remarkable avenue for initiating intimate conversations as it affords one additional time for thoughtful contemplation before articulating their desired sentiments. In this manner, you have the ability to kindle the interest of your partner well in advance, be it minutes, hours, days, or even weeks prior to your physical proximity. You will experience a significant accumulation of sexual tension that, upon finally being united, will result in an intense display of sparks.

The objective in Zone 1 consists of creating such a vivid and stimulating image within your partner's consciousness that it becomes indelibly imprinted. This image will gradually develop over time, much like the infusion process of tea submerged in hot water. Slowly the pictures and ideas will release until the idea has seeped into every crevice of his thoughts. Your significant other will exhibit unwavering admiration towards you. Immersed in the profound essence of your sensuality.

Your inherent sensuality will permeate their every thought and dictate their every action. He will desire the presence of your physical being, the sensation of your touch, and the intimacy of your kiss. You are the sole resolution for this tension. This will evoke a sense of longing and attraction in your partner, even in your absence. Once he is afforded the opportunity to meet you, he will inevitably find himself incapable of controlling his emotions. The greater the level of tension, the more profound and fervent the ensuing sexual experience will become.

Recall an instance in which you experienced a strong desire or longing for a particular item or experience. The idea consumes your thoughts, and your physical being yearns for it. Your sole preoccupation revolves around the acquisition of that particular object. It could potentially be a culinary item or perhaps a musical composition that persists in one's mind. The sole means of appeasing the yearning is by consuming the food or listening to the song. It is necessary to alleviate the tension.

This is the method by which you can incite such an intense level of excitement and arousal in your partner that he will reach a point of climax. Similar to enticing a famished canine with a tantalizing bone, your partner will find themselves utterly incapable of resisting the allure you exude. He will experience it throughout his entire being. He will desire you so intensely that he will be willing to undertake almost any means necessary to attain you.

The following illustrations can be employed via text messaging, telephone conversation, or electronic mail. This will ignite the passionate desires from any remote location. Employ these illustrations in situations where you and your partner are physically separated. Experience the intensifying connection of desire as it gradually escalates, reaching a point of undeniable culmination for both parties involved.

The aforementioned chapter, entitled "Utilizing Text Messages for Remote Stimulation," presents a meticulous procedure for transmitting explicit text messages. At that location, you will discover a comprehensive array of advice and strategies that will equip you with the necessary tools to commence your exploration of the art of Erotic Discourse through written communication. At present, your task primarily entails perusing the provided examples as a means to gather ideas and inspiration. Once you are prepared to commence, you may proceed to the text message instructions provided further along in this book.

Illustrations via electronic means such as text messaging, telephone communication, or electronic mail.

Will you be arriving shortly, or should I prepare myself by dressing appropriately again?

If you were present at this moment, where would you initiate physical contact with me initially?

If you were in close proximity to me at this moment, where would you prefer me to initiate physical contact with you?

I am constantly preoccupied with contemplating the course of action that I intend to undertake upon our rendezvous this evening.

I am in need of rest, yet I find myself unable to quell the vivid images of the actions you could engage in with me, were you to be present.

My thoughts are consumed by you, and I fervently desire your presence within me.

If you were present in this moment, I would engage in various unfavorable actions towards you.

It seems plausible that you have endured a protracted day. I would like to offer you a therapeutic massage this evening in order to alleviate the accumulated tension you may be experiencing. Kindly inform me of the specific areas on your body that require the most attention for therapeutic massage.

I am willing to do anything in order to experience the pleasure of your fully aroused phallus within me. Anything.

I am desirous of making physical contact with a particular region of your anatomy at present. Does it evoke a similar sensation within me?

I find myself currently drenched and unsure whether to engage in self-stimulation or await your presence.

Yesterday night, you appeared in my dream...The memory of it still arouses me.

What will be your initial course of action towards me post-dinner this evening?

I am unable to stop thinking about your firm masculinity. I deeply long for your presence at this moment, so that I may savor its essence.

I've been so bad. I am unable to refrain from engaging in self-touching. It is advised that you promptly join me and engage in sexual intercourse.

I long for your presence at this moment, so that you may witness my self-engagement.

I long for your presence, as it would grant me the opportunity to engage in close proximity with you.

I require your firm and immediate assistance at this moment. Please come over here and give it to me.

Today, my schedule is quite packed with tasks, yet my thoughts remain preoccupied with the desire for your intimate presence.

I am currently removing my undergarments, and the strong arousal that you evoke in me has caused them to adhere to my intimate area.

I kindly request your presence to witness the level of moisture I am currently experiencing.

I desire your immediate presence within me at this moment.

Whenever I close my eyes, vivid thoughts arise wherein I envision you tightly gripping my hair and engaging in passionate intimacy.

I am unable to cease ruminating on our most recent intimate encounter and the exceptional pleasure I experienced while having my legs entwined around you.

I desire to experience the intense presence of your erect organ within me.

When I shut my eyes, I envision you firmly positioning me across your thigh and administering a forceful strike to my posterior. I can discern a nearly palpable sensation.

I desire to orally stimulate your penis to completion, until the entirety of your ejaculate is contained within my oral cavity.

I desire to experience your ejaculation internally.

I would appreciate it if you could strongly consider filling my intimate area with ejaculate.

I derive immense pleasure from experiencing the act where you release your ejaculatory fluids onto my facial region.

I request your immediate attention and assistance.

Please refrain from causing delays and engage in intimate activities with me in a vigorous manner.

I am uncertain if I can continue to wait for you for an extended period of time; therefore, I am considering engaging in activities independently. Wanna see?

I request your presence to attend to a matter of personal nature. I need it now.

I recently engaged in manual stimulation of my intimate area and am experiencing heightened lubrication. May I undertake the task of sampling it on your behalf?

What Is The Optimal Timing For Engaging In A Conversation With My Child?

A significant number of parents express concern regarding their children, particularly when the children start raising queries pertaining to matters of sexuality.

As an involved parent, it is crucial that you ascertain the optimal occasion to engage in a conversation with your child regarding this matter. It is imperative that your child acquires a comprehensive awareness of the realities pertaining to human sexuality from an early stage.

In accordance with this, it is incumbent upon you to ensure that you possess an ample reservoir of knowledge, particularly with regards to matters pertaining to reproductive activities. Rest assured that by employing this approach, your child will gain a thorough and enhanced comprehension of human sexuality.

Within this platform, you will have access to a variety of invaluable resources that will significantly contribute to enhancing your understanding of accurate information pertaining to sexual education. Utilizing these resources will facilitate your ability to discuss avian and insect reproductive education with your offspring.

The Optimal Destinations for Acquiring Knowledge Regarding Human Sexuality

There is a plethora of exceptional resources accessible in the present era, designed to aid you in acquiring comprehensive understanding of matters pertaining to human sexuality. If you are desirous of discussing matters pertaining to sexuality with your offspring, it is imperative that you first acquire accurate and comprehensive knowledge and information regarding the subject.

The Media

In contemporary society, the majority of adolescents and youths are consistently exposed to explicit sexual content and imagery across various media platforms such as films, radio broadcasts, television programs, and publications.

Based on research findings, individuals are initially exposed to aspects of human sexuality through the portrayal of sexual themes in television media.

Rather than comprehending and acquiring the significance of sexual responsibility, a majority of adolescents and young adults are overwhelmed by perplexing messages propagated by idealized and sexualized figures portrayed in the media.

It is imperative for parents to engage in dialogue with their children regarding the content they are exposed to in the media.

A key factor contributing to the impracticability of media filtration lies in its pervasive presence in our surroundings.

The most effective approach to initiate a conversation about human sexuality with your child involves engaging in shared television viewing experiences and subsequently engaging in thoughtful discussions on the various intimate situations they may encounter.

In addition, you may highlight select advertisements and elucidate their intended messaging for the target audience.

It is essential to bear in mind, nevertheless, that media extends beyond television.

In recent times, the internet has experienced a significant surge in prominence within the realm of entertainment, emerging as a pivotal medium that enjoys widespread consumption on a daily basis. It has garnered recognition as an indispensable source of media for the majority of individuals.

Furthermore, it is imperative to engage in a meaningful conversation with your child regarding the presence of video games that encompass explicit sexual content.

Furthermore, it is possible to utilize online resources to provide assistance in educating your child on matters related to their sexuality. Furthermore, one may consider accompanying individuals while they utilize their laptops to peruse the multitude of sex education websites that are presently accessible.

Pornography serves as a noteworthy illustration of the type of online content that your child may inevitably encounter.

It is advisable to educate your child regarding the prevalence of pornography viewing, especially among teenage boys. Nonetheless, it is crucial to underscore the importance of explaining to them that pornography can cultivate impractical expectations concerning genuine sexual experiences, most notably pertaining to women's conduct, inclinations, and physical attributes.

Additionally, it is noteworthy to mention that establishing an emotional bond holds significant importance in the context of sexual relationships. While it is important for your child to understand and explore their sexuality as they grow, it is equally crucial to instill in them the importance of refraining from engaging in sexual activities during their younger years.

Peers

Adolescents and young individuals engage in conversations pertaining to sexuality with their peers as a means of seeking emotional support and moral reassurance. Conversely, peers disseminate inaccurate information pertaining to matters of sexuality.

The dissemination of sexual misconceptions is widespread among many social circles, making it imperative to remain cognizant of this phenomenon.

In adolescent and teenage discussions concerning sexuality, the predominant topics frequently pertain to strategies for preventing pregnancy, engaging in multiple sexual relationships, and pursuing sexual endeavors.

Furthermore, these deliberations may encompass the act of making or mocking evaluations regarding attitudes and behaviors of a sexual nature, consequently giving rise to unwholesome and perilous conduct.

Educators in Schools

The education on sexuality and sex is not provided in all universities or educational institutions. Sexual education courses are also offered at certain educational institutions.

However, they fail to provide comprehensive sexual education to their students. Consequently, there are also educators within the school system who provide factual information on sexuality but overlook the accompanying psychological aspects.

Based on research findings, a proportion of adolescents express dissatisfaction pertaining to the sex education provided at their schools due to its inability to encompass the emotional dimensions and complexities associated with human sexuality.

In contrast, a limited number of establishments offer more substantial support in expressing desires related to sexuality and addressing matters concerning relationships.

It is of utmost importance to strategically select an opportune moment to engage in discussions pertaining to the topic of human sexuality with your child. Through the utilization of these exceptional resources, you can acquire additional knowledge on initiating a conversation of a sexual nature with your child.

Discussing topics related to sexuality and other matters with one's child tends to create discomfort.

Nevertheless, it is imperative to bear in mind that as your child matures, it is essential for them to be cognizant of and at ease with this matter to prevent unforeseen circumstances, such as early parenthood and beginning a family prematurely.

How to compose an alluring piece of writing

Many women encounter difficulty when trying to generate ideas for seductive messages to send to their male partners. The majority of young women tend to overanalyze this particular procedure. Allow me to impart my methodology for generating an extensive repertoire of suggestive expressions. Rest assured, with these techniques, you will never encounter a dearth of creative concepts.

Could you kindly provide guidance on effectively communicating provocative content to one's partner in a manner that is appreciated? It is advisable to employ the five senses, namely touch, sight, smell, sound, and taste, as a reliable guiding principle.

Here are several prompt illustrations:

I am feeling profound physiological responses in response to your presence. I hope you would have the opportunity to physically make contact with them.

*I wish I could feel your cock right now.

I have a strong desire to behold your rooster.

What is your opinion on my appearance, dear? (after sending him a sexy picture)

*I sprayed some of my perfume in your lunch bag so you'll think about me :)

I am currently expressing my discomfort or dissatisfaction on your behalf.

My feline companion exudes a pleasantly fragrant aroma. You're causing me to become quite damp.

I desire the opportunity to listen to the allure of your voice in this moment.

I have an intense desire to experience the flavor of your lips.

I am desirous of consuming your poultry.

Okay, now that we have discussed the fundamental aspects of eliciting a physical response, let us shift our focus towards my proprietary three-step approach to cultivating heightened attraction over the course of the day.

1. Start out slow. Wouldn't you prefer that your partner demonstrates a more respectful and considerate approach

towards intimacy, rather than hastily proceeding with no regard for your comfort or consent? That concept remains consistent in this context. The act of engaging in sexting primarily revolves around cultivating a sense of heightened sexual anticipation. The heightened sense of expectation greatly amplifies the intensity of the eventual sexual experience.

Allow me to present you with a selection of appropriately crafted introductory text messages of a suggestive nature:

I am unable to cease pondering over your existence.

I thoroughly enjoyed our time together last night. Let's do it again.

I desire the sensation of your lips meeting mine once more.

I found myself drenched upon waking this morning.

2. Instigate playful banter with him, but do so modestly. It is often stated that men are less inclined toward women who engage in excessive teasing behavior. Ignore that. They thoroughly enjoy it!

Generate an element of intrigue and obscurity. Allow his mind to contemplate the actions you have planned for him this evening.

Please consider sending him these text messages:

If only you could witness my current attire.

*Guess what I'm doing?

I am currently adorned in the attire that you particularly favor...

May I inquire as to who has displayed inappropriate behavior today?

Please accept my apologies for the typographical errors. Regrettably, typing with only one hand presents a considerable challenge.

3. Go full XXX. Once you have captured his attention and ignited his desire, it is appropriate to gradually become more direct in your text messages (as there is no need for excessive circumspection at this stage). Indeed, we are delving into mature/age-restricted content here.

When you are aware of his genuine interest and heightened sexual desire, employ these text messages to intensify the passion between you two: "

I desire your presence within me.

I kindly request that you remove my dress...

I desire to consume your avian appendage.

You greatly arouse me and create intense sexual desire.

I intend to exert significant effort during our physical encounter this evening.

I intend to provide you with heightened pleasure and bring you to a state of intense climax.

By employing these three steps, I assure you that he will be enthusiastically inclined to engage in the intimate act with you that you desire.

In conclusion, I would like to provide a final recommendation to wrap up this chapter. Strive to integrate shared humor or individual recollections. A simple approach to engaging in explicit conversations is to recount and discuss cherished moments of past intimate experiences. You may even feel an inclination to revisit or replicate those cherished memories.

Nostalgia possesses significant influence, therefore, anticipate and equip yourself to exploit its potential!

Prohibited Practices In The Context Of Sensual Language

If one experiences apprehension when it comes to engaging in explicit conversation, they may assume that it entails evading numerous pitfalls. However, it is rather straightforward to comprehend. Do refrain from displaying skepticism if you believe they are glaringly evident. You will be pleasantly astonished by the simplicity with which these errors can be made if one is not adequately prepared.

Avoid discussing personal relationships or individuals who are not directly pertinent to the conversation.

This will not elicit arousal in your partner. If one were to allude to the familial background of either individual, including oneself, it would have detrimental consequences for the entire affair. Do you experience feelings of arousal when envisioning your spouse's parents during moments of intimacy between you and your spouse? Most probably not, right? Any mention, no matter how slight, concerning her attractive younger sibling is likely to lead to unfavorable consequences.

An imperative rule of utmost significance is to refrain from mentioning any individuals of the opposite sex unless expressly requested by your partner. It is the most expeditious means of instilling insecurity within them. Please be aware that certain individuals may experience arousal when they perceive that others desire them and reciprocate those feelings. However, I must emphasize the importance of refraining from engaging in such behavior unless explicitly requested by your partner.

Please refrain from using technical vocabulary or inappropriate language.

A single word has the potential to utterly disrupt an atmosphere of sensuality. Please be aware that engaging in explicit language serves to enhance the ambience and conjure vibrant mental imagery in the mind of your significant other. The straightforward implication of a term has the ability to rapidly diminish the atmosphere. Do you think you would still experience sexual arousal if your partner expressed, "The weight and texture of your hands resemble that of a gorilla, and they provide a gratifying sensation on my physique"? It is an unpleasant sensation, is it not?

Although the aforementioned example may appear absurd, it remains an undeniable truth that a significant number of individuals employ inappropriate language during sexual encounters. Clinical vocabulary such as "vulva" does not elicit an erotic response. While expressing admiration for your partner's genitalia, employing such terminology may give an impression that it has been directly extracted from a scholarly anatomy textbook. Refrain from utilizing esoteric terminology that may impede comprehension for your counterpart. It is imperative to avoid any potential confusion or distractions that may interrupt their focus and engagement towards your collective endeavor.

The use of juvenile language is generally discouraged too. Referring to breasts as "jugs" or "hooters" does not possess an inherently alluring quality.

Naturally, these considerations do not hold true if one is engaged in a role-playing scenario.

Say It Clearly

Confidence is key. Make every effort to avoid stuttering or speaking with excessive softness. Making errors in your grammar may become uncomfortable, especially if your partner has a strong emphasis on their mastery of the English language. The ultimate objective is to effectively convey your intended message and prompt your partner to contemplate all the points you put forth. If their attention becomes fixated on the manner in which your statement was delivered, it indicates a misstep occurred somewhere along the way.

If occasional stuttering occurs, it is advisable to allocate time for practicing speech in front of a mirror. Don't feel silly about it because your efforts will guarantee a better experience. This will additionally aid in reducing the likelihood of verbal stumbling.

If your voice is excessively soft and low, it is recommended to cultivate the habit of articulating with a resonant and well-projected voice derived from your diaphragm, rather than relying solely on your throat. Please try to speak more quietly. To assess whether you are employing diaphragmatic speech, position your hand at the center of your chest and observe if it produces vibrations while you articulate. If one is unable to articulate loudly, direct your efforts towards enunciating distinctly.

Try and Avoid Repetition

There is no necessity for you to commit numerous phrases to memory in order to achieve proficiency in engaging in provocative conversation. It is indeed quite commonplace to experience a temporary lapse in recollection during instances where one is engrossed in the present situation. If one finds admiration in the melodic quality of a phrase, there might be an inclination to reiterate it frequently; however, it is preferable to exercise restraint and avoid such repetition whenever feasible. The repetition of such discourse may diminish the impact of a particular expression.

To address this matter, acquire a broader range of knowledge to expand your repertoire of expressions. This is where harnessing one's imagination proves most advantageous. Numerous phrases can also be located at the conclusion of this literary work. In the event that you experience anxiety, endeavor to commit to memory a minimum of five phrases while exerting utmost effort to ensure their seamless delivery.

Don't be complacent. Merely because one has achieved success with a particular phrase does not imply that it should be consistently relied upon as the default choice of sentence for every circumstance. Constantly seek new expressions that can be utilized to generate passionate and intense experiences. Ensure that the content remains current and up-to-date.

Know the Tone

Ensure that your manner of conversation remains entirely suitable to the present circumstances. This highlights the significance of thoroughly acquainting oneself with various forms of explicit communication and discerning their appropriate situational usage.

There are numerous individuals who would be deterred if you were to abruptly engage in explicit discussions of sexual nature while partaking in a meal at a sophisticated dining establishment. Conversely, if engaging in vigorous and intense physical intimacy, it would not be opportune to express admiration for their gentle complexion and their wit. Please ensure that your discourse remains appropriate and aligns with the appropriate tone of each given moment.

While acknowledging your fondness for explicit and provocative language, it must be recognized that its frequent use is inappropriate. Please ensure that you gradually progress towards the designated timeframe instead of immediately immersing yourself in the task.

Please refrain from fabricating information spontaneously.

One should confine oneself to expressing ideas that appear authentic, but this does not grant permission to spontaneously create everything. Experienced thespians are required to familiarize themselves with scripts. Hence, it would be advisable for you to attempt the same. While it is possible for a select few individuals to adeptly improvise every sentence they utter, such skills are not universally possessed. It would be advantageous to acquire a repertoire of expressions or, at the very least, possess a preliminary notion of one's intended utterances.

If you attempt to generate ideas spontaneously, your attention will be diverted towards that task, leading to increased susceptibility to distractions. It is highly probable that you will find yourself expressing something awkward or inadvertently humorous. Engage in the repetition of expressions that appeal to you until they have become effortlessly assimilated into your speech.

Your companion will greatly appreciate it.

Strategies For Interacting With Women In A Variety Of Settings

You should engage in conversations with women with the same level of respect and courtesy as you would when conversing with any other individual. The reason behind this is that women are just like any other individual. They are individuals who are similar to us. Despite her unparalleled physical attractiveness, every woman is merely an ordinary individual with identical fundamental desires and requirements as the rest of society. Typically, the issue encountered in conversing with women is our tendency to become reticent or excessively venerate them, thereby projecting a submissive and feeble image of ourselves. In the event that you have encountered difficulties in communicating with women, this chapter will provide an overview of several essential aspects that it would be prudent for you to acquaint yourself with, in order to avoid the misstep of inadvertently sabotaging a potentially favorable outcome.

Be unconcerned with approval. Typically, women are inclined towards men who possess distinct aspirations and exhibit a conscious determination towards attaining them. An alternative way to express the same idea in a formal tone could be: "An effective method to convey such a disposition is to forgo seeking approval in conversations and instead employ assertive and self-assured language." This behavior does not imply being uncouth, disregarding the contributions of other individuals in the conversation, and monopolizing the speaking opportunities of the woman. Instead, it is advisable that you express your thoughts with confidence and clarity. In the event of being subjected to ridicule, refraining from an abrupt modification of one's perspective solely to align with the dissenting party is advisable. In addition, refrain from indulging in sycophantic endorsement of the assertions made by others. If someone, particularly the woman you seek to enchant, utters a statement that conflicts with your views, simply express your dissent. Not intending any form of impoliteness, but as one would expect from a mature individual.

Express romantic interest. Maintaining alignment with the concept of displaying confidence and purpose, if you possess a romantic attraction towards a woman (which is the main focus here), do not hesitate to openly communicate your feelings to her. Masking oneself with clichés and insincere affability is clearly disingenuous; your intent in approaching a woman at a nightclub was not to find a chess partner. She will hold your honesty in high regard.

In the event that she lacks interest in you, she will plainly express her disinterest, thereby allowing you to proceed towards a more receptive individual. Once again, it is crucial to emphasize that employing crude or straightforward language is not advisable. However, it is essential that you articulate your interest explicitly through your choice of words.

Highlight both the positives and the negatives. While engaging in conversation with a woman, there may arise an inclination to express admiration through the bestowal of compliments. She might indeed merit such attention, however, it is likely that she has been subjected to discussions of this nature since her adolescence. It is acceptable to offer her compliments, but you may also choose to acknowledge some of her shortcomings. If she is wearing an unattractive outfit, kindly inform her. Kindly ensure to express it with a lighthearted, playful demeanor. Inform her of your disapproval of her attire, while clarifying that your intention is not to be unkind. Once again, she will demonstrate appreciation for your sincerity.

The most effective approach to communicate with a woman is by practicing sincerity, straightforwardness, and self-assurance.

Inform her of your genuine thoughts, allowing her the opportunity to either accept or reject you based on your authentic self. And should you engage in such discourse with her, it is highly likely that it will result in the latter outcome.

Optimal Approach to Initiating a Conversation With a Lady

I possess an uncomplicated two-step methodology that shall resolve all of your concerns.

The formulated procedure is as follows: Engage in observation, and proceed thereafter with questioning.

"Please permit me to provide an explanation:

Step 1 – Exercise Observation – It is imperative to cultivate a heightened sense of attentiveness when traversing external environments. Not only will it enhance your conversational skills, but it will also enrich your life and enable you to perceive things that most individuals overlook.

When one adopts a keen observant attitude, they gradually discern minute details about her that often elude the average man. Establishing a distinct persona and cultivating favorable rapport with her are of utmost importance when crafting an initial impression. To stand out from the rest, it is imperative that she perceives you as unique and singular, as this perception will grant you continued presence in her life.

Here's a little secret. Women attend to their hair, nails, makeup, coordinate their attire with their handbags, and so on, for two distinct purposes. They desire to appear aesthetically pleasing and experience a sense of contentment. If individuals perceive their appearance positively, it contributes to their overall sense of well-being. When men experience a positive emotional state, they are inclined to engage in conversation with women.

Thus, women endeavor to present themselves in an aesthetically pleasing manner in order to capture the attention of men. It is as straightforward as that. Regrettably, the majority of men do not.

Take note of certain aspects pertaining to her appearance - her hairstyle, manicured nails, eye makeup, choice of blouse, and overall body language. Additionally, evaluate whether she appears to be anticipating someone's arrival. These factors will greatly influence the trajectory of your forthcoming conversation.

Observe your surroundings. Various events and circumstances in your surroundings, including ambient temperature, olfactory sensations, peculiar individuals, and the presence of a person engaged in conversation with her, might be occurring. Perhaps based on her nonverbal cues, it seems that she may not be displaying any interest. An effective strategy would be to calmly sit adjacent to her and behave as if you have a longstanding acquaintance. After his departure, kindly inform her that she appeared to be in need of assistance, and subsequently resume the conversation.

Step 2 - Question. By posing open-ended conversation questions instead of using an interview-style approach, one can effectively manage and direct an entire discourse. You begin by inquiring about matters derived from your observations, patiently awaiting her response, expanding on the subject, and pursuing it to its fullest extent. If this initiates discussion on another subject, that would be excellent! In instances of silence or unoccupied time, kindly inquire about another observation that you have encountered.

Hello, I must say I quite admire your choice in footwear. Could you direct me to a location where I could potentially acquire a pair of said items for the purpose of gifting them to my sibling on her birthday?

How to engage in playful and affectionate communication with a woman whom you find yourself drawn to

It is highly advisable to initiate a conversation with casual discourse when interacting with a girl you are fond of. Engage in conversation with her regarding general topics such as academics, her social circle, her family, and her personal pursuits. Do not rush her. Maintain a tranquil and composed demeanor in her presence. Exercise restraint in bestowing an excessive amount of compliments upon her. She may perceive that you are feigning it. It is imperative to consistently direct your actions towards progressing from a cordial acquaintance to a close friendship, ultimately culminating in a profound bond of love and longing.

Commence by embracing a sense of levity and acquire the skill of being clever, endeavoring to interject some humorous anecdotes.

This would contribute to her increased comfort levels during interactions with you. The majority of young women combine both intelligence and confidence. Therefore, convey to her the impression that you consistently uphold your commitments and possess unwavering confidence in yourself. In the event that you express yourself in a manner that is not perceived as intended, it is advisable to subsequently incorporate a light-hearted remark to transform the situation into a jest.

One must exude self-assurance as a pivotal aspect of engaging in the act of flirtation with a young lady.

Engaging in non-verbal communication can be employed to express romantic interest towards a lady. Body language is an essential but often overlooked part of communication. The clothing selection is just as crucial as body language when it comes to flirting.

Engaging in flirtation entails maintaining proximity to her without invading her personal space.

The placement of two chairs in close proximity to one another is precisely the ideal arrangement required for that particular moment. Exercise caution in initiating conversations. Extend to her the same opportunity, too. In the event of an extended period of silence during your conversation, consider sharing a brief anecdote with her. Additionally, endeavor to actively engage in attentive listening.

Discover her hobbies and preferences, such as her taste in music, authors she enjoys reading, and so on.

Engage in conversation with her regarding these matters. In the event that you are experiencing difficulty in generating discussion topics, consider initiating the conversation by employing an opener such as "How has your day been?"

Praise also assumes a significant role.

The beauty of a woman serves as her valuable possession. Frequently, when she desires to capture a gentleman's attention, she will proudly exhibit it. Commend her, yet exercise restraint in your admiration. If her intentions are sincere, she will reciprocate your flirtation with heightened intensity. This should be regarded as an indication of acknowledging your flirtatious actions.

You may also initiate flirtation by presenting gifts.

Exercise patience with your beloved lady. Attempt presenting her with small tokens such as a yellow rose and gradually progressing to a red rose. Stuffed animals are frequently favored by young girls. A modest serving of coffee can also greatly enhance your endeavors in the art of flirting.

Another effective method of showing interest is to provide emotional support and offer a comforting presence by extending a shoulder for her to lean on.

Do not cause her to become emotional, but if she expresses the need to share poignant experiences from her life, demonstrate empathy and provide comfort. Make an effort to assist her in resolving issues. Please refrain from excessive interference. She will arrive at your location once she is prepared. Assure her of your constant presence and support. One can effectively enhance her mood by initiating an unexpected, stimulating conversation.

Engage in minimal activities such as maintaining eye contact.

Once you are captivated by her gaze, you can consistently discern if she harbors any inclination towards you. When initiating a conversation with a lady, it is important to consistently observe her eyebrows. If upon immediate elevation, the eyebrows are promptly accompanied by sustained eye contact and a smile, it is likely that you have obtained the affirmative indication to proceed.

How to easily obtain dates with women

Be Witty.

You should possess the ability to engage in conversations with them. You are required to utilize your intellectual faculties and cognitive abilities. They are intimidating. You simply need to prioritize establishing a substantive dialogue with them. You must endeavor to impress them with your intellect. You must endeavor to engender in them a perception that you do not experience intimidation in their presence. It is essential for you to create a favorable impression. If you perceive her to be intellectually astute, it is imperative that you engage in further literary pursuits. You must acquire additional knowledge. You must peruse literature that aligns with her interests. In this manner, when she inquires, you possess the knowledge of what to articulate.

Build Up That Confidence.

Do not allow your insecurities to consume you. It is imperative that you enhance your self-confidence. Now, how can one achieve such a task? It's simple.

One can commence by cultivating an appreciation for oneself. You may delineate all the commendable characteristics that you possess. You will come to recognize that you possess a multitude of valuable assets. It is important to bear in mind that one's insecurities tend to become evident through their posture, gait, demeanor, and communication. When one adopts a slouching posture, it indicates discontent or dissatisfaction with one's own self. It is crucial that you consciously endeavor to enhance your self-esteem periodically. You may initiate the process by engaging in activities that bring you pleasure.

Be The Casanova.

You have the potential to embody the qualities that they have been deeply desiring for. Please refrain from expressing her beauty upon sighting her. Convey to her something unique and unfamiliar. Compliment her attitude. She will perceive that your interest in her is not solely based on her physical appearance. Furthermore, you can propose the notion of providing transportation by offering to drive her back to her residence. It would be greatly appreciated if you could perform this kind gesture. You have the ability to engage in actions that can greatly impress and captivate her.

When all other options prove unsuccessful, consider engaging in contrary actions.

Yes, it is ironic. However, it is possible that the footwear may not be suitable for her. You have the option to present yourself as either the rebellious individual or the irksome figure that she finds bothersome. It requires immense courage to undertake this endeavor as some individuals may not succeed in their attempts.

You may exhibit a superficially unkind demeanor towards her. You possess greater capabilities compared to her. Perhaps that is what she requires. She requires a partner who surpasses her abilities and is not intimidated by her.

The Psychological And Physiological Factors Of Erotic Communication

Sensory stimulation does not solely lead to arousal. As per scientific investigations, the utilization of seductive expressions, whether spoken, whispered, or exclaimed, possesses the intrinsic ability to elicit neurochemical responses within the brain, thereby amplifying states of arousal. The neurotransmitters present in the brain during the act of engaging in explicit dialogue and sexual activities are specifically dopamine, known as the neurotransmitter associated with feelings of happiness, and oxytocin, the neurotransmitter responsible for fostering an enhanced sense of emotional connection with one's partner.

You are familiar with the sensation that occurs when your significant other gazes at you with purpose and longing. Your natural instinct starts to kick in. You seem to have a singular focus on one aspect...sexual activity. The sexual response cycle can be divided into four distinct phases, namely excitement, plateau, orgasm, and resolution.

Excitement

During the commencement stage, the release of serotonin takes place. It serves as a neurotransmitter that is recognized to elicit feelings of happiness. When an individual experiences excitement or arousal, the dilation of their pupils occurs. It is an indication that your autonomic nervous system is functioning at elevated levels. Additionally, it signifies your inclination towards another individual. Hence, in previous eras, women employed a substance to be applied to their eyes with the intention of dilating their pupils, a visual cue intended to allure potential suitors. The phenomenon of dilated pupils in fact enhances a man's level of attraction towards a woman. Furthermore, the secretion of adrenaline occurs during the phase of arousal. The heart rate commences to accelerate. An increase in blood flow occurs in the genital region. A male individual's genital organ undergoes tumescence. The clitoris and labia minora of a woman experience swelling. Males undergo scrotal constriction and testicular inflammation. Male individuals undergo the release of fluid intended for lubrication. Women's genitalia also experience an increase in vaginal lubrication. The release of dopamine leads to an elevation in one's sexual drive. All of your experiences become heightened. You have now attained a plateau.

By establishing a profound connection between the cognitive and physical aspects, one amplifies the experience of sexual intimacy to a heightened degree. There are numerous means of arousing a partner without any physical contact to their genital area during the phase of heightened excitement. Allow your warm exhale to be felt by your partner...rest assured, your lover will become mesmerized. Engaging in auditory expressions of pleasure can provide significant arousal for your romantic partner. Furthermore, it provides a source of intellectual stimulation for you. The act of producing melodious sounds can stimulate the energy centers located in your throat region. Nevertheless, it is unnecessary to feign the role of a pornographic performer. Allow your expressions of discomfort to arise organically.

Plateau

Building upon the initial sense of excitement, there is a subsequent elevation in important physiological markers such as heart rate, blood pressure, respiration, and muscle tension. Norepinephrine, akin to adrenaline and exerting an effect of elevating blood pressure, is discharged upon stimulation, thereby heightening sensitivity in the genital area. Muscular contractions might manifest in the feet, hands, and facial regions.

Orgasm

Amidst the climax, the muscles in the pelvic region undergo contractions. The female's uterine muscles and the male's penile base undergo coordinated rhythmic contractions. The considerable accumulation of nervous and muscular tension is discharged simultaneously and involuntarily as highly enjoyable surges. Men ejaculate their semen. Females also have the capacity to encounter ejaculation. At the moment of climax, there is a peak in the oxytocin level within your body, which is commonly referred to as the "love hormone." Researchers posit that oxytocin is pivotal in fostering trust and intimacy within romantic partners.

Resolution

Typically, sexual arousal tends to diminish during the phase of resolution. The contraction and swelling diminish. Certain women may potentially regain the ability to enter the orgasmic phase. Nonetheless, males experience a refractory period, during which they are unable to achieve orgasm. Men have the capacity to exercise patience and subsequently engage in further sexual activity. If a couple refrains from engaging in sexual activity at that time, they may opt for cuddling, which prompts the release of oxytocin (referred to as the love hormone). This hormone fosters further development of trust and intimacy between individuals.

All stages may incorporate the inclusion of explicit verbal expressions. As an illustration, acts such as engaging in explicit conversations, engaging in virtual sexual encounters, and expressing sexual desires verbally, both face-to-face and at the onset of a sexual encounter, are commonly observed during the phase characterized by heightened arousal. The plateau phase may encompass directives that communicate the desires and feelings of each partner towards one another. During the climax stage, partners may engage in explicit communication wherein one describes the intense sensations they experience as they reach orgasm, such as expressing the sensation of release or the feeling of their partner's presence. Finally, the resolution phase can consist of dirty talk related to how good the partner made them feel. We shall subsequently delve into specific instances, progressing from gradually integrating suggestive language to eventually exploring more explicit forms of dialogues.

You Are An Exceptional Kisser."

Can this contribute to enhancing intimacy during foreplay, while also providing gentlemen with a performance-driven approach, wherein positive feedback boosts their enthusiasm?

Your arms possess considerable appeal.

Unlike women, men do not often receive physical compliments, therefore expressing your admiration for his physique can greatly enhance his self-esteem and confidence.

"I Need YOU."

Given that the cues indicating female arousal are significantly more subtle compared to those of males (as it is readily apparent when he is being flirtatious), he eagerly seeks any form of validation that you are attracted to him.

Please place your mouth on my bosom."

Extending a provocative invitation reminiscent of Christian Dark showcases your confidence, authority, and a desire to intensify the encounter, all of which are highly appealing. Any intense desire yearns for the proximity akin to Frantic Libs ("I wish to engage with your ___." "Obtain access to my ___.")

I greatly appreciate the manner in which you finish my tasks.

Penetrating you is one of the most enjoyable moments of sexual intimacy for a gentleman, as he experiences a distinct sensation of making a significant impact upon encountering your vagina for the first time. Illustrating the impression experienced upon his arrival draws attention to your astute perception of his considerable size and formidable hardness.

"Ohh GOD."

This phrase imbues sexuality with a sense of being forbidden and unimaginable, while concurrently indicating a state of complete bliss.

Deploy it during an exceptionally extraordinary moment.

It is an astounding sensation when you place your penis against me."

Many individuals experience feelings of insecurity regarding the size, shape, or appearance of their wand of enchantment. Therefore, expressing your appreciation for his masculinity enhances his confidence and increases his level of arousal.

F - ME HARDER.

Expanding your sources of motivation beyond your comfort zone by employing words such as "breasts," "vagina," or the derogatory term for female genitalia conveys that you have relinquished your boundaries and allowed primal urges to dominate. To maintain authenticity and avoid giving a fraudulent impression, it is recommended that you use strong language judiciously. Adjust your speech to correspond with your level of enthusiasm, being increasingly explicit as you approach the peak of your excitement.

I greatly appreciate our intimate encounters together.

By attesting to the extraordinary intimacy experienced when lying side by side afterward, you enhance the profound connection between you and your partner, as well as your overall satisfaction. Moreover, considering the fact that his levels of the hormone oxytocin, which promotes bonding, reach their peak after sexual activity, he is yearning for a sense of intimacy and connection.

Speak With Your Partner

Prior to commencing this endeavor, it is imperative to ensure mutual consent and willingness between yourself and your partner. To bear in mind, engaging in tantric sex notably requires the active participation of both individuals involved. If you harbor interest in pursuing this, it is imperative to ensure that your partner shares a similar outlook. A significant proportion of individuals fail to perceive that this is a circumstance which their companion may not be adequately prepared for.

Although I appreciate your enthusiasm for beginning immediately, it is essential to consider the following point: engaging in tantric sex requires open discussion and mutual participation, as it entails a two-step process that must be undertaken collaboratively. If both parties lack interest or fail to collaborate, it will not come to fruition.

Furthermore, in the event that you are engaging in tantric sexual practices while your partner does not partake, it will result in an imbalance where only one individual experiences intense orgasms and desires a more leisurely pace, whereas the other may seek a more vigorous approach. It appears somewhat inequitable, doesn't it? The primary challenge encountered in engaging in tantric sex in any alternative manner is the inability to achieve desired outcomes and successful implementation.

And it should not prove difficult to persuade your partner to give it a try. Ultimately, the objective is to cultivate a greater sense of emotional closeness, enhance the quality of intimate experiences, intensify the level of desire and imbue the relationship with an overall sense of enjoyment.

Obtaining your partner's agreement regarding this matter should be relatively straightforward, as it is highly likely that they will derive enjoyment from the introduction of new spices and diversification alone.

Make the Necessary Arrangements for the Deceased's Body

Preparing the body is a good thing to do with tantric sex because it takes time. Frequently, individuals fail to recognize that tantric evenings can impose a certain level of physical exertion. Furthermore, it frequently enhances one's sense of self-worth. You will enhance your bodily sensations and achieve a state of holistic well-being.

When you experience a state of physical well-being and the environment is appropriately arranged, it will induce a tranquil state, resulting in the most exceptional intimate experiences.

What are several activities or tasks that you are capable of performing? Primarily, if one does not aspire to invest extensive hours at the fitness center or exert excessive effort in honing physical fitness, one may opt for the practice of yoga.

Yoga is an excellent option that you will have the privilege to engage in. It is a highly significant development that will greatly enhance your overall experience.

Furthermore, yoga not only enhances flexibility, but it also encompasses postures that can positively influence one's sexual experiences. Certain items are specifically designed to enhance the experience of tantric intimacy and may be incorporated into such encounters. Additionally, it aids in the process of reestablishing energetic balance.

It is inferred that the energies within your body emanate from the spinal region. Hence, it is imperative to ensure that your back remains in a state of relaxation, avoiding any hunching or slouching. It is important to ensure that the activity is performed in a manner that does not cause harm to oneself and avoids any adverse physical impact on the back.

Nutritional Recommendations

Shifting our attention to the realm of nutrition emerges as the subsequent sphere of concentration. Dietary habits are indeed equivalent in importance to physical fitness, and they also play a significant role in enhancing tantric experiences during nights. Adhering to a diet does not necessitate adhering to a convoluted menu crafted by a self-proclaimed expert. Rather, it entails adopting a nutritional approach that significantly improves your well-being. The most optimal approach would involve the cultivation of healthy habits and the implementation of moderation. Endeavor to refrain from excessive indulgence as you approach the forthcoming tantric evening. It is advisable to abstain from consuming substantial meals prior to engaging in tantric sexual activities, and refraining from excessive alcohol consumption is also recommended.

It is advisable to maintain adequate hydration, while exercising caution and avoiding excessive consumption of water as the designated time approaches. This is because you aim to maintain a heightened level of passion, and although restroom breaks are inevitable, you do not want them to disrupt the overall experience.

Furthermore, I recommend searching for detox recipes that prioritize safety. Consider seeking products or services that are highly regarded by users, demonstrating satisfaction, as well as those that have received feedback indicating areas for improvement, allowing for comparative analysis between the two groups.

Do not seek reviews that are excessively positive as well. That's because, happy reviews are faked, but the negative ones aren't either. However, it is imperative to give due regard to safety considerations as well. If you are experiencing a medical condition that is impacting your capacity to adhere to a specific diet, it is advisable to also conduct thorough research on the potential adverse effects associated with it.

It is advisable to limit snacking and, in the event that you do indulge in snacks, it is essential to exercise caution in choosing your food options. There are numerous options available to consume that are nutritionally beneficial and promote good health, while there are equally numerous options that should be limited or avoided. Examine all of these carefully to enhance your comprehension, while also refraining from excessive indulgence in them. Considering the circumstances, is it truly necessary to indulge excessively in those cookies? Probably not.

Unwinding the Physical Self "Soothing the Body "

Prior to embarking on the practice of tantric sex, it is advisable to endeavor to achieve a state of bodily relaxation. Promoting body relaxation holds great significance as the absence of relaxation may induce fatigue and potentially lead to health issues due to heightened stress levels. Following a displeasing day, even in the absence of significant accomplishments, it will appear as though you have engaged in a formidable struggle and emerged defeated, much like encountering a bear.

It is crucial to prioritize not only the physical relaxation of the body, but also the relaxation of the mind. Psychological stress has the potential to compromise the efficiency of your immune system, thereby creating a favorable environment for the proliferation of bacteria and viruses.

Acquiring the ability to unwind is a feasible endeavor; however, it is crucial to bear in mind that aimlessly drifting through life in a state reminiscent of a Zen-like trance is ill-advised. It is possible that you are residing within a persistent state of stress, which often becomes the prevailing condition for numerous individuals. Frequently, individuals are unaware of the extent of their stress, and the financial obligations, social pressures, and strategies for managing stress often contribute to the breakdown of relationships. This concept holds significant importance as tantra facilitates the establishment of an intimate connection that transcends the boundaries of mere physicality and encompasses a profound emotional and spiritual union for numerous individuals.

Frequently, the notion of relaxation can be challenging to grasp. It is conceivable that enduring stress management techniques may pose challenges for you. However, engaging in activities such as taking a nap, enjoying a refreshing shower, or watching a lighthearted film can undoubtedly offer assistance. Meditation holds great intrinsic value; however, it often goes unnoticed and requires one's mindful acknowledgement of personal stress levels, followed by dedicated efforts in self-preparation. If you are experiencing a certain level of dissatisfaction with your appearance, perhaps allocating approximately half an hour each day towards engaging in physical activities such as walking or exercising could prove beneficial. It imparts a sense of emancipation to you in its unique manner. Additionally, maintaining a relaxed state will significantly enhance your ability to engage in tantra, ultimately enabling you to fully embrace and integrate its teachings over time.

Appropriate Attire Selection" or "Choosing Suitable Garments

Certain individuals believe that it is necessary to don excessively fitted and alluring attire. No, I would suggest opting for attire that is spacious and allows for freedom of movement. Additionally, it would be beneficial to select an outfit that promotes feelings of comfort and boosts your overall mood. Certain individuals will engage in wearing garments that symbolize specific deities or originate from the eastern culture. It can facilitate the incorporation of tantra artistry within the confines of the bedroom.

Nevertheless, it is imperative to prioritize personal cleanliness and emotional well-being prior to commencing tantra practice.

Primarily, attend to the cleanliness of your teeth and hair prior to commencing any other task. This is an expedient and uncomplicated method to significantly enhance your self-assurance and facilitate your actions.

Certain individuals prefer to partake in a customary pre-bathing ritual, although it is not obligatory. You should ensure the establishment of a certain level of structure, along with a specific intention to foster a connection that is sufficiently strong, yet not sufficiently intimate as to engage in sexual activity at this stage. It is recommended that you engage in mutual cleansing practices, employing non-sexual methods and utilizing scented soaps and oils. This engenders a sense of anticipation and constitutes a mutually enjoyable experience with the other individual.

It is advisable to engage in activities that cultivate a sense of anticipation for both parties involved. This will, consequently, prove advantageous for the both of you, and will furnish a dignified and skillfully crafted experience with your partner.

Establishing Your Environment

It is advisable to establish an ambiance by incorporating rituals into sexual activities and ensuring that your environment is appropriately arranged. The majority of individuals prioritize incorporating an abundance of white elements within the space, for example through the inclusion of pillows, candles, and soothing music. You are advised to undertake this action with the intention of creating an atmosphere that enhances the significance and intimacy of the sexual experience.

Many individuals tend to hastily enter the bedroom without making a conscious effort to create an ambiance. However, if your intention is to create a lasting impression for all participants involved, I would highly recommend considering the option of embellishing it. Soft, sensual music will help bring forth a better, more intimate experience between both of you. Music has a profound impact on sexual experience, particularly when soft, sensual melodies are employed. This enhances the intimate encounter by fostering a deeper connection, promoting feelings of contentment, and ultimately contributing to overall well-being and happiness for all involved individuals.

Exhale deeply!

Prior to commencing, it is imperative that you take a moment to consciously inhale and exhale in a manner that positively impacts your well-being. This method provides an effective means of achieving mental tranquility and promoting relaxation. What you ought to do is inhale deeply through your nostrils, allowing your abdomen to expand with air, and subsequently exhale. You ought to take note of the outward movement of your abdominal region. That phenomenon is the result of your diaphragmatic respiration, which necessitates your utmost attention and commitment in order to achieve this particular breathing technique. Upon exhalation, one should observe the abdomen gradually reverting to its usual dimensions.

Should you encounter any difficulties with this task, it is recommended that you visualize the downward movement of the pelvis while directing the breath towards the floor. It is advised to practice this activity multiple times prior to engaging in it during sexual intercourse, in order to develop a sense of automaticity and fully reap its benefits.

Engage in Therapeutic Massages

Finally, before you have sex, you should try massaging. These massages need not be of significant duration; however, it is advisable to alternate between the individuals enjoying the leisure activity and those providing it. You may wish to request your partner to massage your feet momentarily, followed by granting them the freedom to engage in any activity of their choosing for a brief duration.

Do not hesitate to provide the necessary feedback during each turn. It is permissible to communicate to your partner areas in which they can improve, as this will assist them in better fulfilling your desires.

This is a predicament commonly encountered by a majority of couples. By engaging in a conversation with the individual, you will have the opportunity to effectively ascertain your desires. Effective communication is a necessary skill that individuals must comprehend as an essential component. The manner in which you collaborate serves as an excellent means for acquiring knowledge. You will have the opportunity to effectively communicate your desires to your romantic partner, and reciprocally, they will enlighten you about their own preferences, fostering the creation of an optimal and mutually satisfying sexual encounter.

It is advisable to take note of the tactile sensations imparted by their hands, the manner in which they make contact with you, the inherent sensuality of this interaction, and subsequently, attain a state of physical and mental relaxation. This will facilitate the enhancement of your capability in managing this matter, ultimately resulting in a state of increased satisfaction and excellence beyond your previous level.

Effective Strategies For Discussing Matters Of Sex, Sexuality, And The Human Body: Guidance For Individuals Of All Generations.

These suggestions can facilitate more streamlined conversations regarding sexual topics with children of all ages.

Articulate concepts using language appropriate for your child's cognitive abilities.

Describe concepts in a manner that aligns with your child's cognitive abilities. For instance, six-year-olds may not require an extensive elucidation on the concept of ovulation; nevertheless, they might be intrigued to learn that women possess minuscule eggs, commonly referred to as ova, which have the potential to facilitate the creation of a human offspring.

It is highly advisable to maintain a concise, objective, and optimistic explanation if possible. Should your child desire further information, they are welcome to return to you. There is no need for you to provide an elaborate explanation all at once.

Younger individuals frequently exhibit a greater inclination towards pregnancy and infants, focusing less on the sexual act itself.

Utilize accurate terminology for anatomical structures.

It is advisable to employ accurate terminology when referring to anatomical structures, such as the penis, scrotum, testicles, vulva, and vagina. It is permissible to employ terms of endearment as well. However, employing the appropriate terminology facilitates the transmission of the idea that discussing these anatomical aspects is indicative of sound well-being and societal acceptance.

If your child possesses a comprehensive understanding of anatomical terminology, they will effectively articulate information pertaining to their body when conversing with you or medical professionals, should the need arise.

Express uncertainty about whether you require

Your child does not necessitate your expertise; rather, your child only requires the reassurance that they can approach you with any inquiries or concerns.

In the event that you face uncertainty regarding a response, kindly express to your child that you appreciate their inquiry, acknowledge your lack of knowledge on the subject, and assure them that you will conduct research to furnish them with the relevant information at a later time. And subsequently, ensure that you do reunite with your child, or alternatively propose the idea of jointly seeking additional information.

Encourage parental participation

In households where there are two or more parental figures, it is advisable for all parents to actively participate in dialogues pertaining to matters of sexuality. When parental participation is present, children acquire the understanding that engaging in conversations regarding sex and sexuality is acceptable.

This can facilitate a sense of ease for children in discussing their anatomy, assuming accountability for their sexual emotions, and engaging in effective communication within close relationships as they mature.

Start a conversation

Certain children may not pose a significant number of inquiries, therefore it may become necessary for you to initiate a dialogue. It would be prudent to contemplate the content of one's discourse in advance and subsequently select an opportune moment to broach the matter. For instance, in the context of television discussions, one might express, "They previously engaged in a conversation concerning pregnancy on the television."

I am curious if you are familiar with the subject at hand. Certain children may feel more comfortable engaging in conversation without maintaining eye contact, thus it may be advantageous to consider having discussions while both you and your child are in transit.

Prepare yourself

You may experience feelings of embarrassment or discomfort when discussing matters pertaining to sexuality, or employing explicit terminology such as 'penis' or 'vagina' in relation to human anatomy. That's OK.

It is advisable to enhance your preparedness by introspecting on your personal comfort levels and subsequently expanding upon them. For instance, should you feel comfortable discussing the lower body region but have reservations about mentioning the chest area, consider initiating conversation by employing the term 'bottom' instead.

Commencing at an early stage with age-appropriate education concerning human sexuality is highly advisable:

Inquisitiveness regarding sexuality is an inherent progression stemming from the acquisition of knowledge pertaining to the physical anatomy. Comprehensive sexuality education facilitates the comprehension of human anatomy and fosters a healthy body image among young individuals. Younger children exhibit curiosity towards the concept of pregnancy and infants, as opposed to delving into the intricacies of sexual mechanics.

Engaging in open dialogue regarding sexuality is integral to initiating open lines of communication with your child. Timely, transparent, and forthright communication between parents and offspring holds significant significance, particularly as one's progeny enters into adolescence.

When a climate of open communication is established, children are more inclined to engage in conversations with their parents regarding various challenges faced during adolescence, including but not limited to anxiety, depression, interpersonal relationships, substance abuse, and sexual concerns.

Commencing a discourse pertaining to sexuality at an early stage and perpetuating this dialogue as the child progresses constitutes an optimal approach to imparting sex education. It enables parents to circumvent the need for a single, potentially distressing conversation with their child during adolescence, when they may have already been exposed to both accurate and inaccurate information from their peers.

These discussions are most conveniently facilitated by drawing upon personal life encounters, such as observing the presence of an expectant mother or engaging with an infant.

When parents talk with their children about sex, they can make sure that they are getting the right information. Parents should be a child's first source of information about sex. Gaining accurate knowledge can shield children from engaging in precarious conduct during their development.

The educational institution premises and the mass communication outlets

It is not advisable for parents to depend on the educational system to provide sex education. Sex education may not be readily accessible, contingent on one's place of residence. In the event that your child receives sex education at school, it is advisable to engage in a comprehensive discussion regarding the subject matter with your child. Inquire about the knowledge they have acquired.

The knowledge that a child acquires through interactions in the schoolyard, friendships, and from la will likely be deficient and potentially erroneous. It could also be perceived as derogatory or potentially perilous.

Despite the pervasive presence of sexual themes and imagery in the media, such portrayals predominantly gravitate towards sensationalism and superficiality. Instances of relationships and sexuality being depicted in a manner that accurately reflects reality are infrequent.

Frequently, matters pertaining to sex and sexuality arise either lacking in context or devoid of any emotional or relational aspect. Additionally, the media frequently underemphasizes the potential hazards of engaging in sexual activities.

Receiving comprehensive sexual education is a more secure and responsible approach than abstaining from providing any form of sex education.

Studies show the more children are exposed to sexual images in the media, the more likely it is they will engage in sexual behaviors at a younger age. Nonetheless, the provision of comprehensive sexual education does NOT result in increased promiscuity. Children who are exposed to comprehensive sexual education within the confines of their households demonstrate a reduced likelihood of participating in behaviors that carry potential risks to their sexual health.

Establishing and promoting open channels of communication with children regarding topics such as sexuality and other relevant matters contributes to their overall well-being and ensures increased safety and security in the future. This does not entail that it will inevitably be effortless or devoid of moments that may cause discomfort.

Adolescents exhibit a penchant for maintaining a high level of privacy. Nevertheless, discussing sexual matters at an early stage enhances the likelihood of adolescents seeking guidance from their parents when faced with challenging or perilous situations.

Remarkable Techniques To Engage In Peaceful Conversation With A Stranger.

1. Go out alone.
Try not to generally go to occasions with a companion, life partner, or relative. Embark on the journey by oneself, thus fostering an obligation to encounter other individuals. If you choose a companion with whom you feel at ease, you are more likely to prolong and engage in conversation with someone you already know you can engage in meaningful discussions with. Similarly, it is impossible to ascertain who your friend will be cognizant of. Envision a situation in which a segment of their acquaintances approach and politely neglect your presence as they proceed to exchange greetings. Regardless, you will inevitably find yourself alone, hence it is crucial that you make the necessary arrangements to adapt to such solitude.
2. Ensure you are prepared to initiate communication.

When you find yourself in a social setting without any assistance, it is prudent not to rely on the assumption that someone will initiate a conversation with you. Individuals are commonly referred to as extroverts due to their propensity for social engagement and proclivity to form acquaintances. Staying in the corner and relying on someone to approach you will not lead to any progress. Do not misconstrue the situation and deem it of significant magnitude. The act of introducing oneself is the principal avenue through which one can establish a connection with another individual. Engage and integrate into the group!

3. Please refrain from engaging in discussions pertaining to the climate. There is no necessity for engaging in a dull conversation. If you choose to commence the dialogue with a frivolous opening statement or an inappropriate comment regarding the weather, it should not come as a surprise if the interlocutor simulates annoyance or departs from the conversation. Phrases

like those restrict opportunities for socialization, as they lean more towards assertive declarations rather than facilitating conversation. Similarly, it is advisable to refrain from using political or religious introductions. Irrespective of the presence of these themes in the information, it remains uncertain as to what might provoke an individual's displeasure. Please refrain from forming opinions about sensitive topics until you have become familiar with the person involved. If you find yourself unable to conceive an intriguing subject independently, simply initiate the conversation with a courteous salutation such as "Hello, how are you?" and observe its progression thereafter.

4. Encourage individuals to engage in self-exploration and meaningful dialogue about their own experiences and perspectives.

A considerable number of individuals prioritize themselves above all else. Even if you have a captivating introduction, one can consistently engage others by inquiring about their own lives, to which they will willingly respond. Inquire about their financial means, inquire about their place of origin, and ascertain their level of education. When engaged in a conversation where individuals discuss their preferences, one can readily observe the manifestation of their authentic personalities. They will be enthusiastic to discuss their extracurricular pursuits, and you may find that you have a commonality in practical terms!

5. However, simultaneously provide information regarding your own background.

It is a common inclination for individuals to engage in self-discussion, yet they also exhibit an inclination to acquire knowledge about others. If you were to interrogate a colleague extensively, it may give them an impression of intrusiveness or being subjected to a relentless cross-examination. Additionally, in the event that you happen to possess similar inclinations, such an occurrence could potentially trigger latent thoughts or information that they had never before considered disclosing. Who could have anticipated that the two of you share a mutual appreciation for collecting stamps specifically from South Africa?

6. Exhibit a courteous demeanor, avoiding assertiveness or coercion. Regardless of the reason for your intention to engage with an unfamiliar individual, it is advisable to avoid exerting excessive pressure. In the event that you harbor a profound fear of disillusionment or feel compelled to fulfill others' expectations, your actions may come across as assertive. In order to engage in a conversation with you, allow them to depart without being insistent and striving to keep their thoughts to themselves. Maintain a relaxed and adaptable demeanor, as this will project agreeableness, thus leading to more fruitful conversations and a higher likelihood of others approaching you.

7. Make an effort to avoid feelings of humiliation in light of your apparent anxiety.

In the event that your voice cracks or your handshake becomes moist, disregard it. If you happen to be a novice performer who possesses the ability to transform it into a jest, broach the subject and elicit laughter in the company of others. In the event that one makes an assumption that induces a decrease in certainty, it is advised to disregard it. Anxiety is a common experience for individuals in certain situations, therefore it is important to overcome it and continue with the progression of our discussion. Make an effort to prevent it from ensnaring or disgracing you to the extent that you feel compelled to depart.

8. Enable your character to shine forth.

Most importantly, act naturally. Provided that you are earnestly endeavoring to engage with everyone, your perceived inconsistency may result in people being deterred from engaging in conversation with you. It is an overwhelming volume of work to conform to all expectations, thus it is advisable to behave authentically and, above all, enjoy oneself. People will take notice and be drawn to your presence.

9. Recognize the appropriate moment to conclude the discourse.

Regardless of whether the discussion concludes in failure or triumph, it is important to be aware of the appropriate time to bring it to a close. If you come to the realization from the outset that you would prefer not to sustain a conversation with someone, endeavor to find a tactful and seamless approach to disengage and seek out an alternative interlocutor. If you have engaged in a satisfactory conversation and established an amicable rapport, kindly inform your newly acquainted individual of your impending departure, but express a genuine desire to reunite on a future occasion. Obtain a contact number or email address and prioritize your personal success in this matter.

Then The What

When pondering over the nature of sexual discussions to engage in with your partner, the appropriate response is to explore a wide range of topics without hesitation or reservation.

You are encouraged to engage in open discussions with your partner regarding any and all topics related to sexuality. However, here are some suggestions to guide your conversation:

For New Relationships

"If you find yourself in a relationship that is still in its early stages, engage in a discussion regarding:

The relationship you want

Are you seeking a relationship that is characterized by a lack of commitment, or are you in search of a relationship that involves strong commitment and dedication?

Is the nature of the relationship platonic or romantic/sexual in nature?

Is the relationship characterized by non-monogamy or monogamy?

Exercising a high degree of precision in expressing your desires can greatly assist in preventing miscommunication and potential emotional distress over time.

STI status

It is imperative for new partners to engage in a transparent discussion regarding their respective sexually transmitted infection (STI) statuses. It is presumed that individuals who have been in a long-term relationship have already communicated and disclosed their STI statuses.

May I inquire about when you last underwent a sexually transmitted infection (STI) screening, and could you kindly share the outcome of said examination?

If you have not undergone testing recently, have your recent sexual partners been tested? What was their status?

Have you ever had a sexually transmitted infection?

Having this knowledge in advance can significantly impact the dynamics of a relationship.

IMPORTANT: It is crucial to disclose any history of testing positive for a sexually transmitted infection (STI) to your partner or potential partners. The greater level of candor and sincerity you exhibit, the more inclined your partner will be to listen to your perspective.

Merely possessing a history of STI transmission does not imply that your sexual fulfillment will be compromised. Please refrain from feeling ashamed; otherwise, your partner will easily detect your sense of shame.

Please make sure to gather as much information as possible about the sexually transmitted infection, covering aspects such as transmission and treatment, in order to establish a strong foundation of knowledge before addressing the topic.

By divulging your personal history, you will create an increased willingness in your partner to reciprocate and disclose their own past experiences.

For Both Emerging and Established Partnerships

Regardless of whether you are in the early stages or a well-established partnership, engage in discussions regarding:

Safe sex

Do you believe it is necessary to employ certain barriers? Would you like to establish a designated word to ensure your safety and well-being? What sexual activities can one engage in without encountering any impediments?

Birth control

Here, you can discuss the most suitable form of birth control for you? Which contraceptive measures do you intend to employ? Are you receptive to the potential occurrence of pregnancy?

Your desires

What sexual activities do you know and want to try with your partner? Are there any experiences that you haven't yet attempted, but believe you have a desire to pursue? Do you possess any desires or imaginings that you wish to openly explore and actively participate in within the confines of your intimate relationship?

Your pleasure

Which touches feel good? In which locations do you experience a particular sense of comfort upon tactile contact? In what manner would you prefer your partner to embrace, gently handle, fondly stroke, or affectionately kiss you? What is your partner's stance on engaging in sole or mutual masturbation?

Your boundaries

Which sexual fantasies are you completely disinclined to pursue? Do you have any bodily areas that you do not wish for your partner to make physical contact with?

Noteworthy suggestion: Within this context, it would be advantageous to construct a Yes-No-Maybe chart. Recommend creating the list in a confidential manner to provide an atmosphere that encourages your partner to express themselves freely.

The affirmation of 'Yes' conveys openness to engage in desirable activities, 'No' indicates aversion towards repetitive experiences, and 'Maybe' signifies a willingness to contemplate and potentially undertake certain endeavors. Once completed, assemble and convene to exchange your lists, engage in dialogue, and undertake further examination.

Frequency

How frequently would you ideally desire to engage in sexual activity? Do you have specified intervals during which you do not engage in sexual activity, or do you have a specific timeframe in mind during which you would prefer to engage in sexual activity? Would you be interested in allocating some additional time for intimacy? Are you experiencing feelings of pressure and desiring a decrease in frequency?

IMPORTANT: It should be noted that this list of topics pertaining to sex is not comprehensive; our exploration has only begun to scratch the surface of the subject matter. These prompts serve the purpose of initiating and stimulating your ideation process.

Should you wish to engage in a discussion pertaining to matters concerning your intimate relationship, please feel free to communicate openly with your partner without any hesitation. Please keep in mind that your partner is a person with whom you envision engaging in intimate activities for an extended period of time. Failing to address the matter would result in enduring silent suffering, as effective communication is necessary for your partner to be aware of your concerns.

Furthermore, it is imperative to emphasize the importance of fostering open communication as a means to engage in discussions about sexual matters, ultimately enhancing both your relationship and intimate experiences.

You have been acquainted with the underlying reasons, location, timing, and essential details; it is now time to delve into the methodology:

Talking About Her First Period

From a technical standpoint, the transition from girlhood to womanhood occurs when a female commences menstruation. Menstruation is indicative of a woman's physiological state, signifying her readiness for reproductive capabilities. Nonetheless, it is widely recognized that a girl of 9 or 12 years of age is, in every facet, ill-prepared to undertake the role of a mother. Similarly, adolescent males may possess the biological ability to procreate, however, they have yet to acquire the necessary capacity to fulfill the duties and obligations associated with fatherhood. This constitutes an additional substantiated basis for advocating that parents adopt an engaged stance in imparting knowledge about puberty and sexuality to their offspring.

As your daughter reaches the threshold of adolescence, it is essential for you to be present and guide her in preparing for this significant biological milestone - her first menstrual period.

Menarche and Menstruation

Menstruation is a significant milestone in the process of female adolescence. Your juvenile daughter may experience feelings of anxiety regarding the onset of her initial menstrual cycle, and the most effective approach to reassure her in this matter is to facilitate her comprehension of the menstrual process. Menarche, in clinical terminology, refers to the initial occurrence of menstruation in girls. The onset of menarche signifies the maturation of all aspects of your daughter's reproductive system. On a monthly basis, it is customary for a woman to experience a menstrual cycle. Fundamentally, menstruation denotes the expulsion of blood and tissue.

The Menstrual Cycle

On a monthly basis, a single ovary produces an egg. The ovum undergoes transit within the fallopian tubes en route to the uterine cavity. In this period, the endometrium of the uterus undergoes substantial proliferation of tissue and accumulation of blood. Upon the occurrence of fertilization between the egg and a sperm, the resultant embryo will undergo attachment to the uterine wall, subsequently progressing towards further developmental stages, ultimately leading to the formation of a fetus. Nevertheless, in the absence of fertilization, the expulsion of the egg, excess blood, and uterine lining tissue takes place as menstrual discharge.

This reproductive process will commence during the onset of puberty and persist until the onset of menopause. During gestation, the menstrual cycle ceases. There can be variations in the menstrual cycles of women. Certain individuals may experience a menstrual cycle lasting 28 days, whereas others may encounter cycles lasting 24 or 35 days. The duration of the menstrual cycle is contingent upon the ovary's ability to generate and release an oocyte.

Certain females may experience a consistent menstrual cycle, while others may encounter irregularities in their monthly periods. Should you have any apprehensions, it is imperative to seek expert advice from a medical professional to acquire further understanding of your daughter's menstrual cycle. The physician can also provide you and your child with information regarding what is considered normal and abnormal with regards to menstrual cycles. They have the ability to suggest alterations to dietary habits or the provision of supplements in order to regulate your daughter's menstrual cycle or reduce discomfort experienced during menstruation.

The Female Reproductive System

Parents should not overly concern themselves with this matter. There is no requirement for you to deliver a comprehensive presentation encompassing all the components of the reproductive system. To effectively educate your daughter about menstruation and reproduction, it is essential to possess a fundamental understanding of the key components of the reproductive system and their respective functions. Acquaint yourself with the primary components of the female reproductive system, namely the uterus, fallopian tubes, ovaries, cervix, and the vagina. If you are able to procure a visual representation, it would facilitate the child's comprehension of the physiological aspects associated with menstruation, sexual intercourse, and the process of reproduction.

Main Components of the Reproductive System

• Ovaries – A pair of elliptical organs responsible for egg production.

• The Fallopian Tubes are a pair of conduits facilitating the transit of eggs from the ovaries to the uterus.

• Uterus - The reproductive organ where the eggs undergo fertilization.

• The cervical region encompasses a passageway that extends from the vaginal opening towards the uterus.

• The vaginal opening functions as a conduit for the expulsion of menstrual fluid, facilitates sexual intercourse, and facilitates the process of childbirth.

CHAPTER 3

DIRTY TALK GUIDELINES

• Ensure that they are interested in it.

When discussing explicit language, exercise prudence as not everyone is receptive to it, and individuals who are not interested may be significantly deterred by it. What are the indicators to determine whether engaging in explicit language is advantageous? The most reliable indication that your use of inappropriate language is well-received is when you receive a reciprocal response employing similar language.

For instance, if one expresses admiration for the intimate connection experienced, and in response, the other person reciprocates with a similar sentiment emphasizing satisfaction derived from the physical union, it can be inferred that one's approach has been successful. Even in the absence of verbal communication, there are often subconscious reactions exhibited such as moaning or alterations in body language. Kindly devote your attention to your partner and observe the successes and shortcomings. To simplify matters, if your partner is engaging in explicit conversation, reciprocate with similar dialogue.

Engaging in explicit communication can be highly beneficial in maintaining the emotional closeness within long-distance relationships. Establish a sense of sexual anticipation through the verbal articulation of sexual matters to one another. Alternatively, consider participating in telephonic intercourse to enhance your sexual gratification.

• Incorporate explicit language into your romantic partnership

What is the most appropriate approach to initiate explicit conversation? Just try it out. Amidst intimate moments, endeavor to express something exceptionally complimentary, yet provocatively enticing. An exemplary instance would be, "An illustration of this would be when you say, 'Your physique stimulates a strong reaction within me.'" The feminine counterpart of this expression is 'Your physique generates immense moisture within me.' I am unaware of any individual who would not appreciate such sentiments being conveyed to them during intimate encounters.

As you develop a greater sense of assurance and ease in expressing yourself, endeavor to venture into unexplored territory. Perhaps at some point you will articulate something negative — it does not signal the culmination of everything. As long as you refrain from crossing the boundaries to the extent that it becomes absurd, such as uttering statements like

'Yes, you perform oral sex, you repugnant individual,' or any similar remarks, you will be in good standing."

• Keep it positive

It is imperative that you consistently maintain a positive tone. Unless there has been a explicit and comprehensive conversation with your partner affirming their consent to engage in negative/degrading experiences.

As an illustration, using a phrase such as, 'Do you find that appealing?' "You possess a rather promiscuous nature," represents a more formal way to convey the same message However, expressing such sentiments as "Do you have a preference for that?" could potentially shift the tone of the statement to a more unfavorable context. "You exhibit behavior that is unbecoming and promiscuous." By using more elevated and formal vocabulary, the statement conveys a similar meaning without resorting to explicit or offensive language. It indirectly suggests that the person in question engages in immoral or inappropriate conduct. Many individuals do find pleasure in experiencing humiliation, but it would be unwise to presume that it is the same for your partner. Inquire with your partner about their desired form of sexual communication. If you have not inquired, it should be presumed that they have a dislike for humiliation."

• It is advisable not to attempt to rectify the situation.

According to Brown, it is important to bear in mind that vulgar language serves the purpose of being explicit. If one attempts to purify it, it assumes a comical facade. 'Your ass looks so good bouncing on my cock' is hot, but "Your buttocks looks so good bouncing on my genitals' is stupid. Keep it dirty!"

• Refrain from procrastinating until you are in bed

Engaging in provocative conversation does not necessarily entail using vulgar language or explicit descriptions. It could instead involve a spontaneous message expressing intense desire, or other methods of creating a mood for future intimate encounters. We have numerous suggestions for engaging in sensual communication if you require inspiration for what to say.

• Modify your explicit language according to your conversation with your partner.

The exchange of verbal and physical expressions during a sexual encounter significantly depends on the preferences and inclinations of one's partner. Please be aware that identical phrases may not yield the same results with every individual. For instance, while referring to your previous partner as 'Mummy' might have instantly aroused her, your current partner may perceive it as an interference to his arousal. Therefore, do not hesitate to modify and refine your intimate communication to suit your present partner.

• Set aside your thesaurus.

A high school research paper provides an excellent opportunity to display one's extensive vocabulary, whereas the bedroom is not an appropriate context for such a display. To avoid sounding unprofessional or kitschy, refrain from mentioning a 'swollen member' or 'engorged mammary glands' if you do not wish to come across as a failed romance novel writer. Additionally, based on scientific evidence, it has been proven that 20% of the population strongly dislikes the term 'moist,' therefore it is advisable to exclude it from your vocabulary.

• Keep it general

Frequently, when discussing explicit matters, it is advantageous to maintain a general approach. This holds particularly true when discussing the physical attributes of your romantic partner. While you may appreciate their ample derriere or well-developed thighs, it is important to note that these physical attributes could be sources of insecurity for them. Reminding them of these features is a guaranteed method of dampening the atmosphere. Rather than discussing specific dimensions and contours, it is advised to maintain a more generalized approach and express sentiments such as, 'I derive immense pleasure from tactile encounters with your physique.'

How Often

Is it Appropriate to Send a Text Message to a Lady?

Determining the appropriate timing and frequency of communicating with women via text poses a challenging dilemma for men, as various divergent opinions on this matter abound. There exist divergent views on the frequency of texting among individuals, with some advocating for constant texting, others discouraging it, while a subset advocates for frequent texting. The issue at hand lies in the challenge of substantiating any given perspective amidst a plethora of viewpoints, as few are supported by verifiable evidence.

Upon conducting research, we encountered a study conducted by WhatsYourPrice.com, encompassing a survey of 1,595 male individuals aimed at assessing their texting behaviors. The research revealed that individuals of the male gender who engage in daily texting exhibit a greater propensity to receive a higher number of replies, experience an enhanced level of response quality, demonstrate superior sexual performance, and display an increased likelihood of committing to a new acquaintance. We know, so what?

Indeed, we possess something of superior quality. The studies themselves indicate that one does not necessarily need to engage in excessive text messaging in order to achieve favorable outcomes. The study, in truth, revealed that the most favorable quantity of text messages is between 10 and 12 per week (equal to one per day), along with a maximum of one response per hour. Therefore, it is unnecessary to communicate with a woman via text message every hour in order to observe desired outcomes.

The outcomes of this study come as no surprise to us, as we regularly receive inquiries from gentlemen inquiring about the appropriate frequency of texting a woman. The reality is that it is contingent upon the kind of relationship you desire to have with her. If your objective is to acquaint yourself with her, it is not imperative to engage in frequent texting. If you desire to sustain her attention for a longer duration, it is imperative to engage in more frequent texting.

Taking all of these factors into consideration, we shall now examine the aforementioned study conducted by WhatsYourPrice.com and endeavor to ascertain the implications of the findings for individuals of average standing such as ourselves. Furthermore, we aim to provide guidance on the appropriate frequency of texting women.

The following are the results of the conducted study:

The findings indicated that male individuals who engage in a lower volume of text messaging per week (specifically, 3-6 texts) tend to receive a higher frequency of replies. Conversely, men who send a significant number of texts on a weekly basis demonstrate an average level of replies. To put it differently, as you increase your frequency of texting women, their responsiveness to your messages will diminish. This phenomenon can be attributed to two factors:

1) A woman may receive a multitude of text messages from gentlemen expressing their interest in her, and as such, she is not obliged to respond to every individual unless they pique her interest in some manner.

2) A woman will receive numerous messages devoid of personalization from individuals of the male gender who solely harbor an interest in her physical appearance, particularly emphasizing aspects such as her physique, posterior, or other bodily attributes. These

individuals exhibit disinterest in acquainting themselves with the woman and hold the belief that by engaging in persistent advances towards multiple women, they will eventually encounter someone possessing additional noteworthy qualities.

Additionally, the research indicated that males who engage in sending a range of 10 to 15 messages per week experience favorable outcomes. The underlying cause for this phenomenon is identical to that which yields positive outcomes for individuals who send a frequency of 3-6 messages per week. Females may find themselves inundated with text messages from gentlemen who lack genuine interest in meeting them, leading them to seek prompt disengagement. Gentlemen who engage in sending a moderate number of 10-15 texts per week generally exhibit commendable qualities such as kindness, respectfulness, genuine interest in the woman, and a preference for concise yet affectionate text messages. Through the avoidance of generic communication methods, they refrain from intimidating the woman with their excessive self-confidence and assertive text messages.

In addition, the study observed that males who exceed a frequency of 15 messages per week demonstrate a proclivity for diminished levels of intrigue and respect within their textual communications. There appears to be a reluctance among women to respond to men who demonstrate excessive effort. Individuals who communicate beyond a frequency of 15 messages per week often demonstrate a proclivity towards

being critical or engaging in
unwarranted mockery towards women.

There exist unique possibilities for
engagement with written
communication, yet it is imperative to
establish a solid foundation for your
relationship with a woman prior to
embarking on such endeavors. One
would unlikely find sufficient time to
engage in all these activities when
initially encountering an individual,
particularly in the scenario where the
interaction originated from an informal
message but ultimately progressed
positively. It is imperative that you
maintain her engagement and capture
her interest until you have the
opportunity to meet her in person.

"Allow us to provide some guidance regarding the appropriate frequency for texting a woman:

1. Minimize the transmission of superfluous text messages, or preferably, make an effort to refrain from doing so. The message communicated to a woman should evoke positive emotions and influence her sentiments in a desirable manner. It is not a matter of eliciting an immediate response from her, rather, it is about sustaining the luster and vitality of the connection for as long as feasible. In the event that she is committed to someone else at the time you come across her message, there exists an opportunity for you to potentially pursue a relationship with her. In the event of her lack of interest, she will disregard your presence and proceed.

2. When engaging in textual communication with a female individual, ensure that it is undertaken with a clear and intention-driven motive. It is advised not to casually send her a text message without a valid purpose or without sharing any crucial information about yourself or your endeavors. She would become irritated if your messages lack meaning and are impersonal in nature. The messages that you send ought to hold significance; they should possess a unique and sincere quality.

3. Please refrain from exceeding a maximum of 10-12 text messages per week. It is unnecessary, and comparable outcomes can be achieved by transmitting 2 or 3 effective messages per week. Achieving favorable outcomes can also be attained by transmitting a

quantity of 10 or 15, provided that you adhere to the aforementioned guidelines. Otherwise, you will not experience success in this regard.

4. Refrain from sending frequent, hourly text messages to a woman. Please refrain from sending a message within a five-minute timeframe following her previous message. It would be appropriate to express your interest in that moment, but it would be better to reserve it for the occasion of your actual meeting with her.

5. Avoid using generic texts in your communication, such as sending messages like "Hey, what's up?" or "How are you doing?" Women possess the ability to promptly discern when a gentleman is exerting excessive effort

and, correspondingly, they may begin to disregard one's presence. Incorporate a brief introduction of yourself within your text message to provide her with an understanding of what to anticipate from the ensuing conversation.

In conclusion, the aforementioned study indicates that one does not necessarily need to inundate an individual with a high volume of text messages in order to demonstrate interest or make progress in a romantic pursuit. There are a couple of options available in order to achieve this objective: reducing the quantity of messages sent while focusing on the quality of each communication. Women are adept at detecting any alteration in your communication patterns, and their response will either be favorable or unfavorable, with no room for ambivalence.

Eight Strategies To Enhance Your Sexual Arousal

In the realm of both literature and film, it can be observed that the depicted characters exude a fervent and anticipatory aura after emerging from their private quarters with the intention of engaging in a sexual encounter. However, it is important to acknowledge that such portrayals do not necessarily align with the actual complexities of these situations in real life.

On certain occasions, there may arise circumstances wherein you delay your entry into the bedroom until your partner has completed the act of undressing, while on other occasions, you might experience distress irrespective of your partner's words or actions.

It is advisable to refrain from engaging in sexual activity if you are not feeling well. But on days when you have sex and feel good, here are some tips to increase your libido.

This chapter examines several prevalent factors contributing to individuals' reluctance towards sexual activity. We further extend our services by providing advice and suggestions aimed at enhancing opportunities for interpersonal closeness.

Factors that could contribute to a lack of positive emotions towards sexual activity

It is crucial to delve into the reasons underlying one's discomfort with sexual experiences in order to effectively address and resolve such feelings. Engaging in various strategies and techniques with the intention of improving your well-being can prove to be exasperating if you fail to recognize your lack of desire for sexual activity.

Several potential causes for diminished or decreased sexual desire may include:

Restlessness

Cultural or religious impact

Depression

Embarrassment or remorse

Hormonal change

The pressures of existence (such as mortality, procreation, or relocation)

Medications

Chronicle of past instances of mistreatment or decline

Issues within the interpersonal rapport

If you are experiencing any of the aforementioned scenarios or have made any of the aforementioned observations and find yourself responding to sexual desire, it is advisable to seek guidance from a medical professional in order to mitigate potential medical and emotional consequences. And relational healing.

8 strategies for engaging in intimate encounters

Now that you are aware of the underlying factors contributing to diminished sexual desire, you are now well-equipped to initiate the implementation of appropriate remedies. If you suspect that your diminished sexual desire may be attributed to a medical ailment, it is advisable to seek consultation with a healthcare professional or specifically, your physician. Nonetheless, in the event that it originates from circumstances beyond your influence, such as stressful situations or fatigue, presented here are a few recommendations to facilitate the rekindling of your sexual desire.

Prioritize self-care "Attend to your own well-being "Ensure your own welfare "Look after your own needs before others'

In instances when my emotional state is unfavorable, I experience a sense of contentment that impedes my ability to derive pleasure from sexual activities. You may experience fatigue, feelings of depletion, or go through phases that are not consistently appealing. All of these factors can potentially influence your inclination towards engaging in physical intimacy.

Commence your journey towards a balanced nutritional regimen and consistent physical activity. Please pause temporarily and allocate some time to include additional information. Research indicates that engagement in physical activity consistently augments sexual drive.

It can often prove challenging to engage with resources in a sexual manner. If an individual engages in excessive smoking or alcohol consumption, there are available resources that can aid them in reducing or completely abstaining from such habits.

Attempt New things

There come instances when individuals may choose not to engage in sexual activity due to feelings of ennui or unease. This phenomenon is particularly prevalent among individuals who have established enduring partnerships. Both of you can enhance the intimacy in your relationship by engaging in new and unexplored experiences. It has the potential to incorporate toys into one's sexual experiences or engage in erotic role play.

Alternatively, you may consider modifying the surrounding environment. Reserving accommodations at a high-end hotel can revive the passion within your intimate relationship that remained undiscovered.

Nevertheless, prior to addressing matters related to sexual intimacy, it is imperative to express gratitude for the emotional closeness shared with your partner. The expression of emotions enhances the level of sexual arousal.

You and your partner will jointly partake in the exchange of physical, emotional, and experiential elements. Engaging in open communication with your partner, whereby you express your desires while attentively listening to their desires, significantly contributes to fostering emotional intimacy and security between the two of you, ultimately promoting physical intimacy.

Allocate time for intimate relations.

A significant number of couples regard sexual intimacy as a secondary consideration after a demanding day. While it may not seem like a fun thing to do, writing down a specific time in your schedule to have sex can make a big difference in your sex life.

Strategizing intimate moments allows for the opportunity to dedicate undivided time to connect with your partner. Additionally, it primes both your physical and mental state in anticipation of the undertaking, affording you the opportunity to relish the experience.

Stress management

Engaging in sexual activity and experiencing pleasure can be challenging when one is under significant stress. Whilst it may be convenient to assert that one should eliminate stressors from their life, there exist specific methodologies that can be employed to effectively regulate stress levels.

Establish a consistent regimen of physical activity, engage in mindfulness practices such as meditation, and cultivate mindful respiration techniques to effectively regulate stress levels and enhance sexual drive.

One of the foremost measures you can undertake to facilitate nocturnal resting. In the event of sleep deprivation, it has a detrimental impact on one's productivity throughout the day, as well as on the quality of rest obtained in the bedroom.

Please remember to unseal your circumstance.

Exhausted and fatigued, confide in your partner. As an illustration, certain individuals derive sexual arousal through the act of engaging in textual communication with a significant other. One can commence by dispatching a letter of gratitude to one's partner.

Sending love messages to your partner increases the emotional connection between the two of you, which can put you in the mood for sex. Perhaps you could engage in light-hearted banter throughout the day and observe the natural progression of the situation.

Some couples enjoy a hot sexting session hour before they have sex. Additionally, you can engage in the perusal of literature or audiovisual materials that explore sensual or provocative themes. If your partner wants, you can turn them on and watch or read together. This can enhance both the inclination for physical closeness.

Make yourself happy

Masturbation can serve as a beneficial means to revitalize one's body during periods of physical discomfort. Regardless of the duration of your relationship, it is indisputable that you possess the most comprehensive understanding of your own body, surpassing anyone else. Take a moment to unwind and settle into a position where you prefer to experience gentle physical contact.

If it is agreeable to both you and your partner, you may consider engaging in the act of self-stimulation while both of you are present in the confines of the room. If you find yourself motivated, you have the option to extend an invitation to your partner.

Modify the schedule for gender assignment

Should you discover that sexual activity with your partner exclusively occurs during nighttime, following lengthy days, this may be a contributing factor to your diminished inclination towards engaging in intimate encounters. Engaging in sexual activity during the nighttime may be perceived as monotonous or unexciting, particularly within the constraints of a hectic lifestyle. Alternatively, prioritize engaging in intimate activities in the morning during the upcoming week.

Engaging in sexual activity in the early morning, following a sufficient period of rest and rejuvenation, can serve as an effective means of enhancing one's sexual desire.

It is completely within the realm of normalcy to experience occasional lapses in the experience of sexual desire. If one's libido is experiencing a decline, it is advisable to invest time in discovering one's preferences and identifying stimuli that elicit excitement towards sexual activity. Do not subject yourself to unnecessary stress. Dedicate time to intimately exploring your own sexual identity whether individually or in the presence of a partner. If one experiences a persistent sexual inclination over a prolonged period, it may serve as an indication of an underlying condition that warrants discussion with a professional of this caliber.

CHAPTER ONE

THE SEXUAL WALL

The Pervasiveness of Sexualized Messages In contemporary society, sexual images and messages have become increasingly prevalent. On a typical day, what is the duration within which you are typically exposed to messages of a sexual nature? Sex and sexuality can be portrayed through various mediums, such as television, music, billboards, print media, the Internet, telephone and communication devices, cable, and cinema.

Approximately four decades past, upon encountering a publication bearing the name Playboy, I experienced an undeniable sensation akin to traversing the realms of heavenly bliss and returning.

Nevertheless, among contemporary young individuals, a Playboy magazine can be deemed as a form of mild stimulation, reminiscent of the experience I had as a youth with National Geographic, which featured portrayals of unclothed individuals from tribal societies. Similar to my own experience, it may momentarily captivate one's attention, although the effect is transient. Merely by activating the computer, children now have unrestricted access to observe explicit sexual conduct at their discretion.

In households where children have unrestricted access to the Internet, a realm of explicit sexual content is just a few clicks away. They have the capacity to witness sexual intercourse encompassing a range of expressions, ranging from conventional to highly unconventional, perverse, and aberrant practices.

Numerous children have the capability to bypass PC Internet filters or employ alternative devices for Internet access, irrespective of their household's possession of such measures. If the Internet is not available, alternative options could include cable television or access to pay-per-view movies. There is an abundance of sexual encounters available for all individuals. Cable television presents a diverse array of sexually explicit content, albeit potentially less provocative compared to the Internet. Additionally, your child's mobile device can potentially facilitate the exchange of explicit photographs among peers, and social networking platforms can host a range of sexually explicit content and communication.

Even if your child is merely in the age range of four or five, it is imperative to deliberate upon the extent of her susceptibility to the impact of televised content. Although she may lack a full understanding of the sexual content she is exposed to, rest assured that she is indeed assimilating it. And it is highly likely that upon commencing her education, she will undoubtedly be affected by the interactions with her fellow classmates.

It is evident that a wide range of electronic and communicative devices can be utilized to procure explicit sexual material.

In addition to these technologies, contemporary children are subjected to numerous alternative means of receiving sexualized content. Pop musicians delve into the subject of sexual relationships and casual encounters, accompanied by songs that contain derogatory and offensive lyrics towards women. This amalgamation offers a captivating range of sexualized prospects within the realm of music. When amalgamated with video, they form a genre that possesses the potential to inundate the senses with captivating narratives pertaining to sex, sexuality, and gender. Print media, such as magazines, novels, newspapers, and various forms of advertising, offer extensive possibilities for sexual depiction. The advantages are further enhanced by the inclusion of peer interactions.

Establishing Protective Measures for the Well-being of Our Youth

I have included a straightforward illustration to aid in your comprehension of the challenges our youth face. Kindly imagine a scenario where your offspring is situated at a table. An extensive assemblage of square blocks, each measuring one inch, envelops the entire expanse of the floor in her vicinity.

Each block represents a message of a sexual nature in some capacity. Perhaps she unintentionally comes across explicit conversations among acquaintances, encounters sexually suggestive content on television, or is exposed to sexually explicit lyrics in a song. It could potentially consist of any content that is sexually explicit or incomprehensible in nature. The presence of sexual content, however, is omnipresent in every neighborhood, exposing one's daughter or son to explicit messages on a daily basis.

A solid object is positioned on the surface of the table before your child for the initial encounter with one of these sexualized messages. Following her second exposure to a sexualized message, an additional block is placed adjacent to the original block on the table. A block is positioned adjacent to the second exposure, followed by subsequent placements in the sequence, until the row spans a length of eighteen inches.

A second block is placed on the initial block in the first row in sequential arrangement. With the advent of each subsequent sexualized message, the pattern perpetuates.

A third row commences once eighteen supplementary blocks are positioned. The construction of a block wall commences.

Have you understood the concept? Take into account the vertical dimension of the wall following a mere 24-hour time span. What is the count of sexualized messages or blocks that would be present on the table in front of your child? Evidently, the correlation between the height of the wall and the age of your child is apparent, as it is logical to assume that an older juvenile would possess a broader spectrum of experiences, thereby being more exposed to sexual themes. In your estimation, how much vertical growth do you anticipate the wall to have achieved within the span of one week?

Might I propose considering this option for a duration of one month? What is the estimated duration of time required for you to complete this task? Could you please clarify your statement regarding the duration of one year? What is the duration of time that has elapsed? If compelled to make an estimation, it is my belief that the uppermost extent of the barrier comprised of sexualized communications directed towards your child extends considerably high above the earth's horizon, surpassing the limits of our perception. Take into account this particular situation: It is highly probable that your child has been exposed to an extensive number of sexualized messages, reaching numbers in the thousands, if not tens of thousands, by the time they reach adolescence. To what extent can we anticipate a proliferation of these sexualized messages that have the potential to inflict harm and stand in opposition to your established principles?

To what extent will these portrayals depict women as sexual objects and men as pursuers of sexual desires? What is the anticipated prevalence of homophobic and heterosexist attitudes? To what extent will the depictions entail engagement in sexual intimacy and activity without consideration for accountability or repercussions? To what extent will a proportion of them portray sexual relationships as unattached to the presence of romantic love?

To what extent do these concepts elude the understanding of your young child, if not totally confounding? From which locations do they originate that would make you feel uncomfortable?

A comprehensive analysis of the Sexual Barrier

Doesn't this elicit a slight tremor in your spine? How will the appearance of such a wall, filled with provocative cues, change as your child enters puberty and starts to express their sexual thoughts

167

and desires, while also being increasingly influenced by their peers?

What will be the extent of its elevation when it occurs? Your offspring is situated in close proximity to an immense barrier displaying sexualized propaganda. As guardians, it is incumbent upon us to aid our children in unraveling that impediment.

What is the current ownership distribution between yourself and your partner in relation to those blocks?

Are the proportionate positive effects of your intimate messages able to counterbalance the detrimental impact they had on your child? Should you fail to assume the role of your children's primary and authoritative provider of sexual guidance, they will readily and effectively receive such information from their acquaintances, peers, and the media. Would you prefer for your child's exposure to sexualized messages to primarily come from the media and their friends, or do you believe it would be more beneficial for them to receive such messages from you?

It is widely recognized that the media and the social circles of our children possess considerable sway in informing and molding their perspectives regarding sex and sexuality. Consistently, study after study reveals that peers and the media consistently emerge as the primary influential sources of sexual information.

The Detrimental Sexual Messages Conveyed by Parents to Their Offspring

However, it is of paramount importance to address you, the parent, as a primary consideration. What type of information or guidance do you impart to your child regarding sexual matters? How many wall blocks in your collection provide uplifting and affirming messages for your child? To what extent have these factors adversely affected your child, contributing to their sense of uncertainty and confusion? Do you instruct your young son to exhibit fortitude, resilience, and physical prowess? Do you grant permission for your nine-year-old daughter to don low-cut tops, short skirts, and apply cosmetics? Are you interested in establishing a friendship with your child, yet encounter challenges when it comes to establishing limits and conveying denial?

Your lack of verbal communication carries significant implications.

During a recent parental presentation at a school, a caregiver of a nine-year-old child relayed to me that her offspring's closest companion possessed an iPad and regularly accessed highly explicit online platforms, subsequently exposing the child in question to objectionable imagery. She asserted that she caught wind of her son discussing the matter and proceeded to engage in a conversation with him regarding it. He had expressed his disgust, albeit noting that it was not a significant matter.

It is within your jurisdiction to prevent the occurrence of this event. Please direct your concerns to the parents of the other boy. It would be imperative for you to discontinue permitting your son to associate with that boy if their perspectives do not align with your own. Then it is essential that you provide guidance to your child in interpreting the explicit sexual material to which they have been exposed.

On one side of the equation, I can comprehend the rationale behind her response. Every caregiver strives to avoid disappointing their child by potentially terminating a friendship. It is evident that she should engage in rational discourse with the parents of her son's friend's child and endeavor to convince them about the seriousness of the situation: it is inappropriate for nine-year-olds to be exposed to sexually explicit content.

It is presumed that they would consent and take appropriate measures to address the situation concerning their child. Nevertheless, in the event that they decline to adhere to her appeals, she may be compelled to apprise her child of the unfortunate news that he will henceforth be prohibited from consorting with his acquaintance. As arduous as this situation may be, it pales in comparison to the perils associated with allowing a child of merely nine years to have access to explicit and sexually-oriented materials on the internet.

Let us examine the multitude of messages that were published on her son's sexually suggestive digital platform, as stated by the parent during the presentation. Undoubtedly, her nine-year-old son has been undoubtedly exposed to explicit sexual behavior, quite possibly on multiple occasions. We are cognizant that he possesses an understanding of his mother's awareness, however, she has not yet articulated her viewpoint. Consequently, numerous hazardous blocks have been added to his wall. The adolescent is currently navigating the challenging realm of highly sexualized visuals independently, while also grappling with the perplexity of his mother's lack of intervention.

In the absence of the guidance and support from a discerning adult, the exposure of young children to excessively sexualized imagery can have a significant impact. Subsequently, in subsequent sections of the book, I shall expound extensively on this matter.

Currently, our only expectation is that his mother will intercede to mitigate the adverse consequences of the obstacles. I am optimistic that she will communicate to her son that witnessing sexual activities is unnecessary, that explicit videos don't consistently present a realistic depiction of adult sexuality, that she will engage in a conversation with the mother of his friend and request her intervention in preventing his friend from accessing and sharing sexually explicit content, that she will remain open for discussion about anything he may have encountered on the iPad, and that she is undertaking these actions out of her deep affection for him.

www.ingramcontent.com/pod-product-compliance
Lightning Source LLC
Chambersburg PA
CBHW051731020426
42333CB00014B/1251